SLEEP NEEDS, PATTERNS, AND DIFFICULTIES OF ADOLESCENTS

SUMMARY OF A WORKSHOP

Forum on Adolescence

Mary G. Graham, *Editor*

Board on Children, Youth, and Families
Commission on Behavioral and Social Sciences and Education

National Research Council
and
Institute of Medicine

NATIONAL ACADEMY PRESS
Washington, D.C.

NATIONAL ACADEMY PRESS 2101 Constitution Avenue, N.W. Washington, D.C. 20418

NOTICE: The project that is the subject of this report was approved by the Governing Board of the National Research Council, whose members are drawn from the councils of the National Academy of Sciences, the National Academy of Engineering, and the Institute of Medicine. The members of the committee responsible for the report were chosen for their special competences and with regard for appropriate balance.

The study was supported by Grant No. 2925-003 between the National Academy of Sciences and Carnegie Corporation of New York and Grant No. 5294-158 between the National Academy of Sciences and the National Institute on Child Health and Human Development, U.S. Department of Health and Human Services. Any opinions, findings, conclusions, or recommendations expressed in this publication are those of the author(s) and do not necessarily reflect the views of the organizations or agencies that provided support for this project.

International Standard Book Number 0-309-07177-1

Additional copies of this report are available from the National Academy Press, 2101 Constitution Avenue, N.W., Lock Box 285, Washington, D.C. 20055.

Call (800) 624-6242 or (202) 334-3313 (in the Washington metropolitan area)

This report is also available online at http://www.nap.edu

Suggested citation: National Research Council and Institute of Medicine (2000) *Sleep Needs, Patterns, and Difficulties of Adolescents.* Forum on Adolescence. Mary G. Graham, ed. Board on Children, Youth, and Families, Commission on Behavioral and Social Sciences and Education. Washington, D.C.: National Academy Press.

THE NATIONAL ACADEMIES

National Academy of Sciences
National Academy of Engineering
Institute of Medicine
National Research Council

The **National Academy of Sciences** is a private, nonprofit, self-perpetuating society of distinguished scholars engaged in scientific and engineering research, dedicated to the furtherance of science and technology and to their use for the general welfare. Upon the authority of the charter granted to it by the Congress in 1863, the Academy has a mandate that requires it to advise the federal government on scientific and technical matters. Dr. Bruce M. Alberts is president of the National Academy of Sciences.

The **National Academy of Engineering** was established in 1964, under the charter of the National Academy of Sciences, as a parallel organization of outstanding engineers. It is autonomous in its administration and in the selection of its members, sharing with the National Academy of Sciences the responsibility for advising the federal government. The National Academy of Engineering also sponsors engineering programs aimed at meeting national needs, encourages education and research, and recognizes the superior achievements of engineers. Dr. William A. Wulf is president of the National Academy of Engineering.

The **Institute of Medicine** was established in 1970 by the National Academy of Sciences to secure the services of eminent members of appropriate professions in the examination of policy matters pertaining to the health of the public. The Institute acts under the responsibility given to the National Academy of Sciences by its congressional charter to be an adviser to the federal government and, upon its own initiative, to identify issues of medical care, research, and education. Dr. Kenneth I. Shine is president of the Institute of Medicine.

The **National Research Council** was organized by the National Academy of Sciences in 1916 to associate the broad community of science and technology with the Academy's purposes of furthering knowledge and advising the federal government. Functioning in accordance with general policies determined by the Academy, the Council has become the principal operating agency of both the National Academy of Sciences and the National Academy of Engineering in providing services to the government, the public, and the scientific and engineering communities. The Council is administered jointly by both Academies and the Institute of Medicine. Dr. Bruce M. Alberts and Dr. William A. Wulf are chairman and vice chairman, respectively, of the National Research Council.

v

Contents

PREFACE   xi

INTRODUCTION   1

ADOLESCENT DEVELOPMENT AND SLEEP   3

ADOLESCENT SLEEP PATTERNS AND DAYTIME SLEEPINESS   4

CONSEQUENCES OF INSUFFICIENT SLEEP   13

IDENTIFYING AND INTERVENING IN CLINICAL SLEEP PROBLEMS   18

CHANGING SCHOOL STARTING TIMES   23

EDUCATING THE PUBLIC ABOUT ADOLESCENT SLEEP NEEDS   25

NEXT STEPS   26

REFERENCES   31

OTHER INFORMATION RESOURCES   34

APPENDIX: WORKSHOP AGENDA AND PARTICIPANTS   35

SELECTED REPORTS OF THE BOARD ON CHILDREN, YOUTH, AND FAMILIES   46

Preface

This report summarizes the presentations and discussion at a workshop entitled Sleep Needs, Patterns, and Difficulties of Adolescents, held on September 22, 1999. The workshop was organized by the Board on Children, Youth, and Families and the Forum on Adolescence of the National Research Council and Institute of Medicine, with funding from the Carnegie Corporation of New York and the National Institute on Child Health and Human Development, U.S. Department of Health and Human Services.

The workshop brought together policy makers, researchers, and practitioners to examine research on adolescence and sleep. Among the questions it addressed were: How much sleep do teenagers need? What are the typical sleep patterns of adolescents? What are the influences on sleep problems and disturbances? What are the consequences of insufficient sleep? Drawing on participants' presentations and discussions, this workshop summary addresses each of these questions. Of necessity, it reflects the particular emphases of the workshop discussions as well as specific statements made by participants during the workshop.

It is important to note that this workshop was an effort intended to take stock of the current knowledge base on adolescent sleep and to highlight key findings from research. Given the limitations of both time and scope, the workshop could not address all issues that are important in this area. For example, the workshop did not explore in depth the social and cultural contexts that influence adolescents and their behavior.

It is also important to note that this workshop report summarizes material presented and discussed at the workshop. Although it references published materials suggested or provided by participants, it is not intended to provide a comprehensive or thorough review of the field. It is our hope that this report will illuminate important issues related to sleep and the well-being of adolescents that deserve further attention and consideration.

This report has been reviewed in draft form by individuals chosen for their diverse perspectives and technical expertise, in accordance with procedures approved by the Report Review Committee of the National Research Council. The purpose of this independent review is to provide candid and critical comments that will assist the institution in making the published report as sound as possible and to ensure that the report meets institutional standards for objectivity, evidence, and responsiveness to the study charge. The review comments and draft manuscript remain confidential to protect the integrity of the deliberative process.

We thank the following individuals for their participation in the review of this report: Missy Fleming, Child and Adolescent Health, American Medical Association, Chicago, IL; Anthony Jackson, Disney Learning Partnership, Walt Disney Corporation, Burbank, CA; Reed Larson, Department of Human and Community Development, University of Illinois, Champaign/Urbana; Richard MacKenzie, Division of Adolescent Medicine, Children's Hospital, Los Angeles, CA; Barbara McNeil, Department of Health Care Policy, Harvard Medical School; and Shepherd Smith, Institute for Youth Development, Sterling, VA.

Although the individuals listed above provided constructive comments and suggestions, it must be emphasized that responsibility for the final content of this report rests entirely with the authoring group and the institution.

David Hamburg
Chair, Forum on Adolescence

SLEEP NEEDS, PATTERNS, AND DIFFICULTIES OF ADOLESCENTS

Sleep Needs, Patterns, and Difficulties of Adolescents

INTRODUCTION

Sleep is not only a biological necessity but also a physiological drive. In today's fast-paced world, though, a good night's sleep is often the first thing to go. The effects of inadequate sleep are more than mere annoyances: they affect our mood and how we perform at school, work, and home and behind the wheel. Lost sleep also accumulates over time; the more "sleep debt" an individual incurs, the greater the negative consequences, according to researchers in the field (Carskadon and Dement, 1981; Wolfson and Carskadon, 1998).

Research on adolescents and sleep has been under way for more than two decades, and there is growing evidence that adolescents are developmentally vulnerable to sleep difficulties. To discuss current research in this area and its implications in the policy, public, health, and educational arenas, the Forum on Adolescence of the Board on Children, Youth, and Families held a workshop, entitled Sleep Needs, Patterns, and Difficulties of Adolescents, on September 22, 1999. Both the board and the forum are initiatives of the Institute of Medicine and the National Research Council of the National Academies.

The workshop brought together researchers, educators, health care providers, and policy makers to review current findings on adolescent sleep. More than 100 individuals attended the workshop, including medical researchers, teachers, parents, and young people themselves. David A. Ham-

burg, chair of the Forum on Adolescence, and William C. Dement, director of the Sleep Disorders Center at Stanford University, cochaired the
meeting. As Hamburg noted in his opening remarks, the workshop offered
an "opportunity to call attention to a very important and, until recently,
neglected problem area." "Adolescence is the time of greatest vulnerability
from the standpoint of sleep," Dement, a pioneer in the field of sleep research, told workshop participants.   Counterproductive adolescent sleep
patterns tend to be viewed as part of the culture of the teenage years. But
according to Dement and other researchers, the need for sleep does not
decrease as individuals go through adolescence (Carskadon, 1982). The
amount of sleep that adolescents get drops precipitously, however, making
it very difficult for them to avoid chronic sleep loss.

Dement asked the workshop participants to consider several questions:
How much sleep do adolescents require? What factors contribute to sleep
loss in adolescence? What are the consequences of chronic sleep loss in
young people? What can be done about it?

Through presentations and panel discussions, workshop participants
addressed these questions. They summarized results from research over the
past two decades on issues such as how much sleep teenagers need and how
much they typically get, the sleep patterns of adolescents, and the factors—
biological, behavioral, and environmental—that influence them. They discussed recent efforts to facilitate meeting the sleep needs of adolescents,
including consideration of later starting times for high schools and efforts
to educate the public, including parents and youth, on the importance of
adequate sleep. Workshop participants acknowledged the complexity of
the issue and observed that additional research on the causes and consequences of adolescent sleep problems is appropriate. Assessing the impact
and effects of changes in policy and practices by educators, parents, and
youth themselves, as well as increased public understanding of the dimen-
sions of the problem, also could advance the search for remedies.

Drawing on workshop participants' presentations and subsequent question and answer sessions, this report summarizes key themes that emerged
from the day's discussions. It is intended as an overview of the issues discussed for an audience of educators, parents, youth, health care providers,
and other interested readers. It is not intended to provide a comprehensive
review of findings from the entire field of research on adolescent sleep. Of
necessity, the report reflects the content and emphases of the presentations
and discussions. It therefore does not provide full details on research meth-

ods and samples or a critical analysis of the strengths and weaknesses of the studies discussed.

It is important to note that workshop participants agreed that adolescent sleep needs and difficulties are complex issues for which there is no single solution. Because the factors that influence adolescent sleep patterns are both biological and behavioral, solutions need to address those processes as well as the constraints on sleep imposed by the practicalities and habits of young people's daily lives. Additional research is appropriate on a number of topics, as outlined later in this report. Research can also further understanding of the links between sleep difficulties and such outcomes as poor school performance, as well as the extent to which biological rhythms affect sleep patterns in teenagers. Viewing adolescent sleep problems from a public health perspective suggests that public education programs and social marketing campaigns related to other health concerns may provide models appropriate in this area as well.

ADOLESCENT DEVELOPMENT AND SLEEP

To provide a background for examining the sleep problems of young people, Robert Blum, professor and director of General Pediatrics and Adolescent Health at the University of Minnesota, reviewed recent research on adolescent development, highlighting new ways of looking at developmental stages. He noted that, historically, adolescent development has been looked at as a discrete phenomenon. Today, that has changed and adolescent development is understood to be heavily influenced by the contexts within which young people live. In short, young people adapt to their environment as the environment adapts to them.

Puberty is a transitional period between childhood and adulthood. During this time of growth and change, young people begin to develop adult reproductive capabilities and their organ systems undergo dramatic changes. The timing of puberty is extremely variable. For boys the age of onset is between 9 and 15, whereas girls may experience puberty at 8 to 16 years of age (National Research Council and Institute of Medicine, 1999). The age of pubertal onset shifted downward in the 20th century in North America and Europe, due in part to public health factors such as improved sanitation and better nutrition.

Accompanying these dramatic physical changes are shifts in cognitive development. During this period, adolescents move from a child's trial-and-error approach to problem solving to more abstract reasoning and skills.

Completing a puzzle, for example, is likely to be done first by arranging pieces mentally before moving them on the board. Adolescents grow in language sophistication as well, as they begin to grasp multiple meanings of words—for example, puns and double entendres.

During puberty, young people also begin to understand and engage the world differently, shifting gradually from egocentrism to mutuality. With the development of mature social cognition comes the capacity to read social cues, to infer what people are thinking based on not only language but also nonverbal signals. This is seen very dramatically at about seventh grade, when young people start becoming socially savvy. For those who fail to develop this capability, the consequence can mean social isolation.

All these changes take place in particular environments—family, community, social—some of which may promote healthy development and others may predispose adolescents to risk. Research on resilience and protective factors, for example, shows that parental connectedness enhances and promotes healthy development in adolescents. Findings also indicate that having fewer children and spacing births two or more years apart provides greater opportunity for family interaction, Blum said. Parental mental health is a significant influence, particularly if there is a history of substance abuse or psychiatric hospitalization. Conflict within the family undermines the security of the home as a place for positive development. "Children need a safe and secure base," Blum said. "There are two places where they can get this: at home or at school. If neither provides safety and security, the potential for trouble exists."

Blum noted that policies also have an influence—policies related to youth employment, for example. Research indicates that working more than 20 hours a week during the school year is associated with a variety of unhealthy and problem behaviors in youth, including substance abuse, insufficient sleep, and limited time spent with families (National Research Council and Institute of Medicine, 1999). Understanding the influence of various policies, including school starting times, is important to the discussion of adolescent sleep issues as well.

ADOLESCENT SLEEP PATTERNS AND DAYTIME SLEEPINESS

Workshop participants heard from a panel of researchers who reviewed findings from the United States and abroad on sleep patterns and problems in adolescents. They discussed findings indicating that the factors contributing to teenagers' sleep loss lie in both the biological and the social realms.

Mary A. Carskadon, director of the E. P. Bradley Hospital Sleep Research Laboratory and professor in the Department of Psychiatry and Human Behavior, Brown University School of Medicine, noted several major trends in adolescent sleep patterns. Data from cross-sectional surveys of students show that, from ages 10 to 17, students' self-reported bedtimes become later and later, on both weekdays and weekends (Carskadon, 1990; Wolfson and Carskadon, 1998). In middle adolescence, rising times become earlier during the week, due largely to school starting times. High school starting times, which typically are earlier than those of middle and elementary schools, have moved to even earlier hours in recent years. Many begin at or before 7:30 a.m., largely due to the timing and availability of school buses. Thus, while sleep needs remain unchanged, Carskadon said, adolescents are spending less time sleeping, and alterations in sleep schedules during the week compared with those on the weekend are becoming more pronounced. This is in sharp contrast to the stable pattern of sleep found in younger children, who get the same amount of sleep during the week as on weekends—an average of 10 hours a night, Carskadon noted.

The effects of restricted sleep on sleep structure, mood, and performance in children and young people have been evaluated under different conditions (Carskadon and Dement, 1981). In a longitudinal study of sleep and sleepiness in young people, researchers assessed children in a summer "sleep camp" laboratory at Stanford University (Carskadon, 1982). Researchers began studying the children when they were 10 to 12 years of age and followed them every summer for 4 to 6 years. Researchers measured their sleep according to the Multiple Sleep Latency Test (MSLT), a standard measure of sleepiness; the test is administered at designated periods throughout the day to determine the time it takes subjects to fall asleep (Carskadon et al., 1986).

In the laboratory the young study subjects wore electrodes that gauged their physiological reactions in sleep and while they were awake. Each night they had the same 10-hour window of time available for sleep, with sleep latency—the time it takes to fall asleep—tested throughout the day at 2-hour intervals. Starting with the hypothesis that the amount of sleep needed would decrease with age to a typical adult 7.5 hours a night, the study assessed the youngsters at various stages of pubertal development to shed light on the issue of sleep needs.

The results showed that the younger children slept 9 hours and 20 minutes on average and awoke spontaneously. As they progressed through adolescence, they continued to get the same amount of sleep, but they no longer woke spontaneously before the end of the sleep window. At midpuberty, adolescents also became sleepier during the day. According to the MSLT, prepubertal and early adolescents were unable to fall asleep in the daytime, but at midpuberty, even with 9 hours and 20 minutes of sleep, daytime drowsiness appeared and worsened. These older adolescents struggled to stay awake throughout the day, whereas the younger adolescents had no problem at all.

A sleep habits survey administered to more than 3,000 Rhode Island 9th to 12th graders revealed that the median amount of reported sleep in this group was 7.5 hours (Wolfson and Carskadon, 1998). A quarter of these students reported sleeping 6.5 hours or less. For two-thirds of the students, bedtime was after 11 p.m. on school nights; 91 percent rose at 6:30 a.m. or earlier. Seventy percent of the teenagers delayed both bedtime and wake-up time by an hour or more on weekends to try to catch up on their sleep. Sleeping late on Saturday and Sunday, however, usually fosters a later sleep onset on Sunday night. Despite this, sleeping in on weekends allows adolescents to pay back some of their weeknight sleep debt, some workshop participants observed.

Influences on Adolescent Sleep Patterns

The various factors that influence how much adolescents sleep cluster into two major areas. One is intrinsic—the biological processes going on internally in adolescents; the other is the external factors—social, academic, and environmental—that play a significant role in their sleep habits.

Intrinsic Factors

Internal processes themselves fall into two types. One is the biological timing system—the circadian rhythms of approximately 24-hour intervals that influence when and how much we sleep. The second is the internal system that tallies the balance of sleeping and waking—the sleep/wake homeostasis system: when sleep is deprived, more sleep is needed. Thus, as discussed at the workshop, "sufficient" sleep can be defined as the amount that satisfies the homeostatic process and is not associated with daytime sleepiness. This is analogous to the daily caloric requirement to maintain a stable weight.

Research findings suggest that changes occur in the "biological clock" during adolescence. As a result, teenagers have a natural tendency to fall asleep later and to wake up later. This is referred to as sleep phase delay. Carskadon described research on college students that restricted their sleep to 5 hours a night for several nights. This study found that daytime sleepiness increased with each night of restricted sleep, indicating the cumulative effect of sleep loss. The research also showed that even with restricted sleep students felt more alert in the evening, encouraging the tendency to stay up late again (Carskadon and Dement, 1981). If additional tests of sleep latency are carried out at 8 and 10 p.m., a student who struggled and dozed through the early afternoon becomes energetic and internally stimulated in the evening, often past midnight.

Another study that looked at the effects of the biological clock did so by examining melatonin secretion. As night falls, melatonin is "turned on," preparing the body for sleep. Toward dawn, it shuts off, as cortisol secretion increases. Carskadon discussed research on 10 adolescents (five boys and five girls; mean age of 13.7) who were put on a fixed sleeping schedule for 10 days at home. Their schedules were checked by sleep logs, telephone calls, and wrist actigraphy (a device worn to measure daily activity levels). They then were assessed in a laboratory setting on a 28-hour schedule that controlled for all environmental and psychosocial influences on sleep (e.g., lights, television, radio). A correlation was found between subjects' melatonin secretion and their stage of development. The results indicated that melatonin onset occurs later in adolescents, making it difficult for them to go to sleep earlier at night. At the same time, the hormone "turns off" later in the morning, making it harder for them to wake up early (Carskadon et al., 1998, 1999).

At the workshop, Carskadon said that more research is needed to determine whether the apparent changes in melatonin secretion found in this study are a primary intrinsic phenomenon. Comparisons with adults and adolescents under the same conditions are required for more definitive examination. "While it may not be an immutable biological process," Carskadon told workshop participants, "it sets the stage for other psychosocial and environmental conditions that make it easier for these adolescents to stay awake." Adolescent development in general, she added, is "a handshake" between biology and behavior, not just one or the other.

The circadian system is governed by the 24-hour alteration of light and darkness. These findings in a laboratory setting in which light and darkness are controlled suggest that the circadian system can be reset with controlled light exposure. At the same time, Carskadon noted that it may take less light to affect this system. An interesting question is whether teenagers' sensitivity to the ambient light they are exposed to in the evening—including from television, computers, and video games—might contribute to this evening arousal (Minors et al., 1991).

Other participants noted that it is not just sleep loss that is troublesome in adolescents but also the enormous variation in their weekday/weekend sleep patterns. While some argued strongly that allowing students to sleep in on weekends was essential for reducing their sleep debt, others pointed out problems: a youngster who gets up at 6 a.m. on weekdays and then sleeps until noon or later on weekends is experiencing "a Washington to Hawaii time zone change twice a week," said Richard Ferber, a workshop discussant. In effect, the body is in a physiologically wrong time zone.

Other studies have examined teens under the conditions in which they normally function. A field study of adolescents with an early school starting time (7:20 a.m.) showed that many had an elevated rate of REM sleep[1] and fell asleep within 5 minutes during morning MSLT tests (Carskadon et al., 1998). "For these kids," Carskadon said, "biological night is 8:30 a.m., when they are in second-period class." The challenges of engaging such youngsters intellectually when they are in the trough of their circadian rhythms was vividly explored by Catherine Colglazier, a teacher in Virginia (see Box 1). In addition to the obstacles to learning, for those who drive to school the increased risk of accidents because of drowsiness is a serious concern.

External Influences

While an inherent phase delay may make it difficult for teenagers to go to bed early at night, other factors clearly play a significant role in the amount of sleep they get. During adolescence, social obligations and opportunities increase, academic requirements become more demanding, and opportunities for work expand. Young people themselves often point to homework as a contributing factor; however, many adolescents actually spend little time on academic pursuits, Carskadon said. Those on the aca-

---

[1]REM sleep is one of two basic sleep states. This type of sleep is indicated by rapid eye movements similar to those that occur in wakefulness and characteristic brain wave patterns. More REM sleep occurs toward the end of the night.

BOX 1 A Teacher's Perspective

Fairfax County teacher Catherine Colglazier described a typical day at her McLean, Virginia, high school, where the doors open at 7:15 a.m. Students come in either fired up on caffeine or straggly and sleepy eyed.

Because McLean High School has block scheduling, she has 90 minutes at 7:20 a.m. to keep students awake and learning through a variety of activities, including SAT preparation, writing, and literature. At 8:30 a.m., no matter how good the teacher is, some kids are dozing off. Why are they so sleepy? Most students in Colglazier's class reported going to bed well after midnight.

One of the issues teachers face in identifying kids with sleep problems is that parents are reluctant to have such a problem be part of any kind of record or referral for their child because it could be misconstrued as a sign of possible drug use. Another reason that adults seem stymied in helping kids with sleep difficulties is that people don't yet know about or believe the research. In many schools, high SAT scores are evidence that young people are successful. While a student may be taking caffeine pills on a regular basis, acceptance to an Ivy League school speaks louder than any concerns teachers or parents might have.

A second issue is money. There are many competing demands on school systems, such as reducing class size and providing competitive salaries. When it comes to devoting substantial funds to adjust school bus availability and scheduling, a change to an earlier starting time doesn't seem to be worth the money.

A third issue is the impact on extracurricular programs. Since the recent tragic shootings in U.S. schools, most school administrators are working hard to provide a range of activities and clubs that make kids feel connected to school, happier, less violent, and less depressed. The young person who wants to create a club for those interested in computer games is just the sort of teenager schools want in their after-school programs. But doing this is difficult if school starts later.

Cultural factors play a role as well. Americans thrive on stress and admire those who are very active. This is reflected in advertisements and movies, and teenagers respond to the popular culture.

demic fast track, however, do devote more time to school work. Many adolescents are involved in extracurricular activities for many hours a week. For some young people in team sports, this may involve 20 hours or more a week. Many coaches help students plan their sleep, but some youngsters report that practice requirements are a significant factor in their not getting enough sleep, according to Carskadon.

All these things take place in an environment in which television, computers, telephones, video games, and socializing with friends are widely available to most young people, often without parental monitoring and regulation of time spent on these activities. Also, the majority of adolescents have part-time jobs, and many work more than 20 hours a week. Beyond 20 hours is considered to be the point at which working becomes problematic for kids going to school (National Research Council and Institute of Medicine, 1998). A 1994 survey of Rhode Island high school students found that 40 percent of 9th through 12th graders worked on average 20 hours a week (Wolfson, in press).

Working is understood to be an important adult role, Jeylan Mortimer, professor, Department of Sociology, University of Minnesota, observed at the workshop. Studies show that all adolescents, both boys and girls, expect to work during a good part of their adulthood (Mortimer et al., 1999). As noted earlier, adolescence is a time when young people are projecting themselves into the future, and some believe that working encourages "planful competence," a capacity to think about opportunities, potentials, and interests and to plan for desirable outcomes in the future. Working also fosters work readiness—the importance of getting to work on time, proper attire and behavior in the work environment, and so on. Parents are very positive about their children's jobs, reporting that their children become more capable in managing their time and money and in developing social skills and other benefits (Mortimer et al., 1999). They recall the place of work in their own lives in encouraging these same positive traits.

There is, however, a case against adolescent work. It involves concerns that working too much draws young people away from school, reducing the amount of time available for homework and families. There is also growing evidence that working more than 20 hours a week during the school year is associated with a range of problems, including poor academic performance, use of alcohol and other drugs, and risk of involvement in sexual activity and delinquent behaviors (National Research Council and Institute of Medicine, 1998).

Working too much also impinges on the amount of sleep young people get. In the Rhode Island study noted above, analysis of sleep to work time revealed that, for every 10 hours worked, students lost 14 minutes of sleep per night. A student who works 20 hours a week loses approximately 3 hours of sleep per week. In the 5 percent of the sample who worked full time, students lost an hour of sleep per night or 7 hours weekly (Wolfson, in press).

International Comparisons

How do young people in the United States compare with those in other countries as far as sleep is concerned? Amy R. Wolfson, associate professor of psychology at Holy Cross College, presented findings from a number of studies that reveal both similarities and differences. It is important to note, she said, that a comprehensive dataset using similar measurement tools across countries does not exist.

Challenges to International Data Comparisons

A number of issues make comparisons difficult across countries. Definitions of key terms, for example, vary greatly. In surveys done outside the United States, researchers discussing sleep latency—the time it takes to fall asleep—generally describe it as insomnia. It is not clear whether this corresponds to what in this country would result in a diagnosis of insomnia. Rather, it may refer to delaying bedtimes as opposed to genuine difficulty falling asleep.

It is also difficult to discern in studies conducted abroad whether total sleep time is based on an average across both weeknights and weekends. Obviously, what is considered a weekend varies. For example, in Israel the weekend is Friday afternoon through Saturday evening, with students returning to school on Sunday. In addition, minimal information exists regarding school schedules, so the research presented at the workshop reflected only what little could be determined about school start times in other countries.

Research conducted in Amsterdam looked at 1,500 12- to 18-year-olds with school starting times from 8 to 9 a.m. (Hofman and Steenhof, 1998). A second study, in Brazil, looked at a small sample of 12- to 16-year-olds with school starting times of 7:20 a.m. (Andrade et al., 1993). A third study, in Taiwan, assessed more than 900 13- to 15-year-olds (Gau and Soong, 1995); because Taiwan categorizes students academically very differently than does the United States, drawing comparisons with this research is particularly difficult. The total sleep time for those enrolled in this study who were in a more intensive academic track was an average of 7 hours per school night; those in the less intensive track slept about another half hour each night.

A self-report study surveyed students in Austria, Belgium, Hungary, Israel, Norway, Scotland, Spain, Sweden, Switzerland, and Wales (Tynjala et al., 1993). Sample sizes in the different countries ranged from 60 to more than 3,000 students ages 12 to 18. Students in Switzerland reported the most sleep, about 9.2 hours a night (summarized over the week) for 15-year-olds. Israeli and Finnish students reported the shortest total sleep time—between 8.2 and 8.5 hours in the 15 to 16 age bracket. Students also slept more on weekends.

Bedtimes varied generally by about an hour in most countries. Hungarian and Swiss teens reported the earliest bedtimes, on average before 10 p.m. In Spain even the younger students don't go to bed before 10:30 p.m. School starting times are between 7:00 and 7:30 a.m. in Brazil; 8 a.m. in Israel; and between 8 and 9 a.m. in Amsterdam (Holland), Finland, Norway, Great Britain, and Spain. Researchers who looked at European data for a World Health Organization study of health behavior noted that teenagers slept longer in countries in which parental control seemed to be more strict (Tynjala et al., 1993). This observation suggests the need for more research on parental involvement in and influence on teens' sleep schedules in this country and elsewhere.

Research in France studied more than 700 15- to 23-year-olds, focusing on the quality of sleep rather than sleep patterns: 41 percent had at least one sleep problem, and that tended to be the need for more sleep and difficulty waking up in the morning—very similar to U.S. findings (Vignau et al., 1997). In this study sample, researchers indicated that psychological distress was highly correlated with sleep problems.

In summary, available findings from other developed countries appear to parallel U.S. data on adolescent sleep, Wolfson said. Youngsters average 7.3 hours of sleep on school nights and 9.2 hours on weekends. The data also show that sleep time has decreased over the past 10 to 20 years.

Culture and Context

Wolfson emphasized that more detailed, controlled study of teenagers' sleep patterns in other industrialized countries could provide important insights into how students in the United States compare to their counterparts elsewhere. She stressed the need for such research to focus attention on the culture and context in which young people are growing and working. In the United States, for example, teenagers work more hours than their counterparts in other countries, as noted above. In other countries as well as the United States, cross-cultural analysis and documentation are clearly needed. Other factors that should be examined are parental roles in regulating adolescent sleep patterns both individually and as part of particular cultural contexts.

CONSEQUENCES OF INSUFFICIENT SLEEP

What are the consequences of not getting enough sleep? How do we measure them? Ronald Dahl, associate professor of psychiatry and pediatrics and director of the Adolescent Sleep Evaluation Center at the University of Pittsburgh Medical Center, reviewed research that responds to these questions.

Descriptive Data

While sleepiness is the most obvious consequence, the effects of insufficient sleep go beyond that to a drive to go to sleep. This includes involuntary napping—called microsleeps—and gaps in processing information and in behaving reliably. How these relate to accidents and risk behaviors is a critical question. We know that adolescence is a time when young people experiment and explore in various domains. Adolescents who are just learning to drive, who are chronically sleep deprived, and who are beginning to experiment with alcohol pose significant risks to themselves and others.

Another consequence is tiredness, a symptom that entails not just fatigue but also difficulty initiating certain behaviors. Students who are tired do not have trouble doing something that is compelling or exciting. Tasks that are tedious, for which the consequences of failure are more abstract, are the issue. Paying attention to information or tasks that are not naturally engaging—like studying for an exam—is much harder to do when sleep is deprived.

The descriptive data about the effects on mood are very clear, Dahl said. People who are sleep deprived are irritable, showing increased anger and lowered tolerance of frustration. The effects relate to both thinking and emotional control and involve an area of the brain related to the prefrontal cortex, one of the last areas of the brain to develop. Development of the prefrontal cortex is not complete until probably well into a person's 20s, yet adolescents must increase their ability to integrate cognitive strategies with emotions, feelings, and drives. According to Dahl, this system is probably most sensitive to sleep deprivation, with potentially very serious consequences.

Experimental Data

From a research perspective, measuring the effects of sleep deprivation on the integration between cognitive and emotional processes is very difficult. Such experiments must control for individual differences, mood, motivation, and so forth. Dahl discussed findings from a pilot study he conducted with 10 adolescents, in which these factors were controlled in a laboratory setting, comparing the youngsters' behavior when sleep deprived with baseline information obtained before they were kept up all night. The research involved a well-established memory task that required subjects to respond when they saw a match for letters they had seen before. Each time subjects must update memory, which gets increasingly difficult as the test goes on. Typically, this working memory task measures cognitive effects. The pilot study added an emotional background to the letters in the form of a series of pictures that have been rated by thousands of people for emotional content. There were pictures associated with arousing positive emotions, such as sports; arousing negative photos, such as a snarling dog; and visually interesting but emotionally neutral pictures, such as a building.

The results indicated that, for a simple memory challenge, sleep deprivation has no effect; those who are sleep deprived and those who have adequate sleep perform in a similar fashion. But when emotional pictures, both negative and positive, are added, the effect of sleep deprivation becomes apparent. Combining the two revealed significant drops in performance when subjects are sleep deprived. This underpins exactly what adolescents are dealing with every day as they try to control their feelings and behavior and make plans related to school and other responsibilities.

Attention and Wakefulness

David Dinges, professor and chief of the Division of Sleep and Chronobiology of the University of Pennsylvania School of Medicine, discussed other effects of sleep deprivation as shown by research at his laboratory. One of these is a drop in attentiveness and a decreased ability to stay awake (Dinges et al., 1997). Impaired by sleep loss, individuals start a task feeling fine. Minutes later, however, heads begin to nod, and the rate of deterioration accelerates. Instead of being able to sustain attention for a 45-minute lecture in a classroom, for example, a student might be able to manage only 3 to 5 minutes. Wakefulness also becomes unstable, and young people experience rapid and involuntary microsleeps and increasing difficulty in staying awake. Reaction times get longer. This may not be serious in some situations, but a 1-second lapse in reaction time while driving a car at 60 miles per hour translates into 88 feet, Dinges said.

Laboratory tests also measured the ability of subjects to pay attention to a routine task. After one night without sleep, wakefulness is unstable, and with every lapse in attention subjects fail to notice input on a simple object identification test. Such unstable wakefulness not only undermines performance—for example, a student missing an important piece of information from a teacher—but it can also be incredibly dangerous—for example, a sleepy driver missing a stop sign, Dinges said.

Learning

Daily loss of sleep accumulates in a linear fashion. For each hour of nightly sleep that is lost, the price is paid in daytime sleepiness. With 6 hours of sleep a night, evidence of poor performance is clear; with 4 hours a night, the lapses increase day after day, Dinges said. Although conventional wisdom holds that individuals can "train" themselves to adapt to less sleep, laboratory tests belie this. Dinges described his research on young adults (ages 21 to 30) in a laboratory setting for 5 days (where they were carefully monitored so that they didn't nap or do something that affected the amount of sleep they got). He said this study showed very similar results regarding lapse rates as those found by earlier research with the Multiple Sleep Latency Test (Carskadon and Dement, 1981). The correlation between those two laboratory datasets collected 16 years apart is very high, which Dinges said suggested the reliability of the finding that chronic sleep restriction has cumulative effects. Subjects also underwent longer tests, up to 20 days, with measurements taken for 14 days at various levels of sleep restriction—8, 6, and 4 hours. They were monitored by EEGs, and their sleep was recorded. By day 5 those with 6 hours of nightly sleep functioned at an equivalent of one night without any sleep. At 4 hours a night, this happened by day 3. Subjects who continue to get 4 and 6 hours of sleep a night progressed into a zone that is the equivalent of two nights without any sleep, resulting in massive debilitation.

Dinges told the workshop participants that his research shows a significant change in the learning curve associated with sleep loss. With 8 hours of sleep a night, subjects get better and better every day at the assigned task. With 6 hours of sleep, the learning curve is gone, and with 4 hours of sleep the negative impact on learning is even more apparent. Dinges noted that these data show that learning itself—that is, the ability to acquire information, retain it, and then use it repeatedly—is altered by sleep restriction. What this research does not show is the individual's subjective state. Even though young people may say they are tired, they can't tell how impaired they are. They may feel adapted to being tired, but performance tests show the opposite. In tests of sleepy subjects at a computer, researchers observed full 30-second lapses in which the computer alarm went off because the subject hadn't responded for a half minute. With 18,000 opportunities to monitor, no subject sleeping 8 hours had a single lapse. With 6 hours of sleep, a quarter of the subjects had a total of 37 lapses, which started to occur on day 7 and peaked on day 14. Nearly half the subjects with 4 hours of sleep had a total of 188 lapses. The first one occurred on day 6, and they peaked on day 13, Dinges reported.

Adolescents who are allowed to sleep in on the weekends may have an opportunity to pay back some of their sleep debt. While this may mean somewhat less sleep on Sunday night, in the view of some participants it is better than no repayment of the sleep debt.

Emotional Response

Adolescence is also a period of risk for emotional and behavioral disorders. Arousal, stress, or distress may interfere with sleep, setting up a vicious cycle in which emotions cause lack of sleep and lack of sleep exacerbates emotions. These emotions are also related to areas of the prefrontal cortex. Dahl discussed long-term research by his group into sleep, neuroendocrine, and biological measures in adolescents who have severe depressive disorders (Dahl et al., 1996). That work indicates that the most significant biological dysregulation appears to emerge during puberty and is particularly prominent around sleep onset. Youngsters with these difficulties have trouble going to sleep, and REM sleep comes earlier in the night. The study measured their cortisol levels every 20 minutes for 24 hours after they were acclimated to the environment. Depressed adolescents showed spikes of cortisol, the stress hormones, before they went to sleep. And even after they were in deep sleep, they still secreted cortisol, Dahl said.

The Social Context

As noted by Blum, puberty may start early, activating new drives, impulses, emotions, and motivations creating new challenges for the cognitive-emotional interface. Adolescents must develop more self-control over behavior and emotions that involve the prefrontal cortex, one of the last areas of the brain to develop. There is no evidence that the front part of the brain is maturing any faster now than it did throughout human history, according to Dahl. Yet the age of onset of puberty has declined, creating an enormous period of vulnerability as young people face the cognitive and emotional challenges of puberty earlier with relatively less cognitive maturity. All this is occurring in a social context today that gives adolescents a great deal of personal freedom, complex choices, and relatively few constraints.

Driving

Automobile fatalities associated with sleepiness alone as well as sleepiness in combination with alcohol use are a major concern. Analysis of data from the National Highway Traffic Safety Administration estimates that up to 100,000 police-reported crashes annually are related to drowsiness (Knipling and Wang, 1995); among drivers age 15 to 24, more than 1,500 fatalities each year are associated with such crashes. (National Highway Traffic Safety Administration, 1999). Research in North Carolina indicates that such crashes tend to be single-vehicle accidents, both for all drivers and for those under 26 (at least those that get codified by law enforcement). Such crashes tend to occur at night, corresponding to the adolescent circadian profile with its afternoon peak in alertness, which may prompt teens to stay out later. They are more likely to occur in males than females (Pack et al., 1995). These accidents are virtually as severe as those involving alcohol; the likelihood of disabling injury or death is similar, unlike the effects of accidents involving seizures or heart attack. In fall-asleep crashes, there tends to be no compensatory response to right the vehicle (Wang et al., 1996).

Caffeine

Many adolescents drink heavily caffeinated beverages. Dinges told workshop participants that the rate of consumption—estimated to be 153 billion ounces a year—has increased dramatically in young people. Teenagers are consuming more coffee than they did a decade ago, as well as caffeinated sodas (The New York *Times*, April 12, 1998). In short, it appears that young people are using caffeine, the most widely used psychostimulant in the world, to compensate for chronic inadequate sleep, Dinges told the workshop.

IDENTIFYING AND INTERVENING IN CLINICAL SLEEP PROBLEMS

The workshop also explored the issue of clinically diagnosed sleep disorders, beyond sleep deprivation, caused by phase delay or behavioral decisions. When clinicians in adolescent medicine see patients, according to Iris Litt, professor of pediatrics and director of the Division of Adolescent Medicine at Stanford University School of Medicine, they begin with a series of questions. Could this be a primary sleep disorder? Could it be related to some physical disease? Could it be the result of, or associated with, some mental illness? Could it be related to substance abuse? Finally, could this be the result of disruptive forces within the family or home situation?

Adolescent Sleep Disorders

Adolescents suffer from a variety of sleep disorders. In the case of classic sleep disorders such as narcolepsy—characterized by sudden and uncontrollable attacks of deep sleep, sometimes accompanied by muscle weakness—the symptoms in teenagers may be very different from adults. In a study of children ages 10 to 13 with narcolepsy, only one in 15 actually exhibited the classic symptoms (Dahl et al., 1994). Sleep-related eating disorder, a rare condition only recently described in some 25 cases, is the syndrome of partial awakening at night followed by rapid ingestion of large amounts of food, with subsequent poor recollection of the episode (Winkelman, 1998).

There is also a constellation of parasomnias—conditions involving partial wakefulness or interference with transitions in the stages of sleep. One of the symptoms in patients with parasomnias is enuresis (bedwetting). Physicians don't often inquire about this problem among their adolescent patients, but when they do they find that it often has continued into adolescence.

Sleep apnea—a condition involving disordered breathing during sleep—is another one of the primary sleep disorders, but it isn't typically considered in the context of adolescence. It is generally associated with obese older persons and infants. Some hypothesize that with the decreased frequency of tonsillectomies in children, more sleep apnea is occurring in adolescents from upper airway obstructions.

The delayed sleep phase syndrome has many of the characteristics of sleep loss described throughout the workshop. Common effects among teenagers with this disorder include morning sleepiness, poor school performance, sleeping in on weekends, and increased REM sleep.

Physical Illness

Among those disorders associated with physical illnesses, one that is fairly common in this age group is infectious mononucleosis. Sleepiness is a primary symptom but not the only one, and laboratory findings help the clinician make the diagnosis with great certainty. More difficult to diagnose is chronic fatigue syndrome, often first suspected by parents. Chronic fatigue syndrome affects more girls than boys. Teenagers with seizure disorders also tend to have poor-quality sleep and are particularly anxious about falling asleep. Not surprisingly, the frequency of seizures and the frequency of sleep disorders are highly correlated. Similarly, patients with asthma tend to have poor-quality sleep, increased incidence of disturbed sleep, and decreased memory and ability to concentrate. When their asthma is brought under control, the quality and length of sleep, as well as their ability to concentrate, improve.

Emotional or Mental Illness

In recent years, anorexia nervosa has become much more common, found in virtually every socioeconomic stratum as well as every ethnic group. Patients with this disorder have an increase in the number of awakenings and of wakefulness after falling asleep. They have what's been described as decreased sleep efficiency and decreases in their slow-wave (non-REM) sleep. Interestingly, there is a correlation between the ratio of weight to height (as measured by the body mass index) and the amount of slow-wave sleep, which tends to hold true for these patients.

As mentioned throughout the workshop, depression is not only a symptom of sleep deprivation but can also be a cause. A number of teenagers who are depressed have disturbed sleep and insomnia. In teenagers, as in adults, many who are depressed don't seek help from mental health care professionals. They will, however, often see their primary care physicians because of sleep difficulties, which can provide an opportunity to diagnose and intervene in the depression. Anxiety disorders, specifically panic attacks, can occur during the day as well as at night. Such nocturnal attacks can contribute to sleepiness during the day.

Substance Abuse

As noted by workshop presenters, smoking has increased significantly among teenagers, especially among young women who smoke to control their appetite and weight as well as in response to peer pressure and other factors. A number of surveys have shown that those who smoke cigarettes have increased problems falling asleep and staying asleep (Phillips and Danner, 1995). They have daytime sleepiness, increased incidence of depression and minor accidents, and, interestingly, a higher consumption of caffeine than nonsmokers. It is not clear whether the sleep problems reported by smokers are related specifically to nicotine or something else in cigarettes or to their associated increased use of caffeine.

No studies of teenagers have examined alcohol use in relation to sleep cycles, but the adult literature clearly shows that alcohol use is associated with truncated or nonexistent slow-wave sleep episodes and longer REM periods (Lands, 1999). Alcohol has been thought of primarily as a problem of teenage boys, but the gender difference has disappeared. Not only have girls caught up, but in certain studies, particularly of binge drinking on college campuses, girls exceed boys in terms of alcohol ingestion. Amphetamine use also is being seen more and more in girls, who take amphetamines because they suppress appetite. When amphetamine users stop using the drug, part of the withdrawal syndrome includes sleepiness as well as depression.

Sexual and Physical Abuse

Rarely discussed in the context of sleep disturbance is the role that abuse might play. For example, Litt discussed a survey of more than 3,800 girls in a nationally representative cross section of schools. The findings indicated that one in five girls in grades 9 through 12 reported that they had been physically or sexually abused. Among those who reported such abuse, more than 50 percent said they were abused at home. More than half of that group said they were abused by a family member. Two-thirds of those abused at home by family members say it has occurred repeatedly (Schoen et al., 1997). Those who evaluate sleep disorders in teenage girls can ask questions to determine how safe teens feel in their beds and homes. Some teenage girls seek care for sleep disorders, creating an opportunity for clinicians to identify their physical or sexual abuse.

Educating Clinicians About Adolescent Sleep Problems

Many workshop participants observed that training for medical personnel was necessary at all levels—teaching sleep medicine to not only medical students but also pediatricians and primary care physicians. The American Medical Association's Guidelines for Adolescent Preventive Services recommend that all physicians who see teenagers should evaluate certain aspects of each young person's history, including parenting, development, diet, fitness, lifestyle, injury prevention, eating disorders, sexual activity, substance abuse, school performance, and depression (Elster and Kuznets, 1993). Litt noted that the guidelines do not include statements about surveying patients to determine the extent of sleep difficulties. While it is important to teach physicians how to identify sleep difficulties, it is equally important to inform them about remedies, beyond prescribing drugs for sleep.

Understanding Adolescent Sleep Disorders

Mark Mahowald, director of the Minnesota Regional Sleep Disorders Center, noted that sleepiness has long been seen as a sign of laziness, boredom, slothfulness, work or school avoidance, depression, and drug and alcohol abuse. Sleepiness in anyone, certainly adolescents, is due to either volitional sleep deprivation or, more importantly from a clinician's standpoint, a diagnosable and treatable sleep disorder. Until sleepiness is recognized as more than a character defect, individuals with diagnosable and treatable sleep disorders may not receive appropriate diagnosis or treatment (see Box 2).

According to Mahowald, parents need to know that adolescents stay up late because they are not sleepy; they sleep in on weekends not to avoid

---

BOX 2 Diagnosing Sleep Disorders

Mark Mahowald described several cases at the Minnesota Regional Sleep Disorders Center. One involved an 18-year-old referred to the center for excessive daytime sleepiness, which began at 10 years of age. Initially diagnosed with a psychiatric condition, the patient was hospitalized at the University of Minnesota Hospital adolescent psychiatry ward for months with the diagnosis of avoidance behavior. Unable to stay awake in class, he had to leave school. Sleepiness ended his academic career, and the same thing happened when he went into the work force. He couldn't stay awake at work and was assumed to be lazy or avoiding tasks and was fired. Formal evaluation indicated he had classic narcolepsy. Consider whether his academic and employment record might have been different if his sleepiness at age 10 had been recognized as a symptom of a medical disease rather than a psychiatric one and treated accordingly.

Another case is that of a 10-year-old boy with a diagnosis of attention deficit disorder and poor school performance who was in special education classes and taking Ritalin. Fortunately, someone in the school system remembered that one of the first symptoms of sleepiness is impaired sustained attention. After a sleep evaluation, he was discovered to have severe obstructive sleep apnea. With treatment came a dramatic reversal in his school performance, and he was able to go without medication.

A 17-year-old was in danger of being expelled for his inability to get to school on time because of oversleeping. When he did go to school, he fell asleep in morning classes. Actigraphy—monitoring by means of a wrist device to measure daily activity levels—revealed a striking delayed sleep phase syndrome. He was awake until 3:00 a.m. because his biological clock did not permit him to fall asleep before then. But he attended a typical high school, which meant he had to get up at 6:30 a.m. He was expelled even after school administrators learned that he had a diagnosed medical problem.

---

morning chores but because they are calling in their sleep debt. Students need to understand that sleep is important. Teachers need to be aware that sleepiness in the classroom is not necessarily related to drug abuse or boredom. Other school officials need to know that true sleepiness is a serious sign and symptom, Mahowald said.

Physicians at sleep centers routinely see adolescents who have been expelled from school because of sleepiness that is in fact due to an unrecognized and untreated sleep disorder. Mahowald pointed out that students are not expelled when they have seizures, asthma, or other medical problems, but that they are expelled for sleeping in class or not being able to get to class on time in the mornings, when the problem may in fact be due to a diagnosable and treatable sleep disorder.

Qualified sleep centers exist in almost every large community in this country. Most have staff available to talk to teachers, school nurses, school psychologists, and school board members. Sleep medicine experts have both an opportunity and a professional responsibility to integrate scientific data and help broaden understanding of sleep problems and their treatment.

CHANGING SCHOOL STARTING TIMES

Among the responses proposed to alleviate adolescent sleep problems, some school districts have considered changing their school starting times. Workshop participants learned of research in the Minneapolis metropolitan area on attitudes toward such a change and preliminary findings from schools that actually implemented later starting times. During the 1996-1997 school year in Edina, Minnesota (a suburb of Minneapolis), the high school day shifted from a 7:20 a.m. start to 8:30. In the following school year the Minneapolis Public Schools changed the starting time from 7:15 to 8:40 a.m. at seven of its high schools. Kyla Wahlstrom, associate director of the Center for Applied Research and Educational Improvement of the University of Minnesota, reviewed early findings from studies of these schools as well as data collected in surveys and focus groups involving key stakeholders, including students, teachers, and parents (Wahlstrom and Freeman, 1997; Kubow et al., 1999).

The schools studied represent different socioeconomic groups and levels of diversity among student populations. In Minneapolis the schools were in an urban, low-income setting with 12,000 students, including a large immigrant population, where half of the students fail to complete high school. Suburban Edina, in contrast, has high socioeconomic levels and about 1,800 high school students. In Edina, enrollment is stable and most students go on to college.

Early findings from studies in these Minnesota schools showed that a majority of teachers reported that a greater number of students were more alert during the first two school periods than they had been with an earlier start time. Slightly more than half said they saw fewer students sleeping at their desks. In Minneapolis, teachers were evenly divided about whether student behavior improved. Edina teachers indicated markedly improved student behavior. School nurses and counselors also reported fewer students seeking help for physical complaints or stress. In Minneapolis schools, both teachers and students reported a drop in the number of students involved in extracurricular activities; later schedules also posed difficulties for some students who worked after school. Edina students and teachers saw no significant change in after-school activities, including work. Wahlstrom emphasized that these were early findings and that both additional data and further analysis are needed on the effects of changes in school starting times (Wahlstrom, 1999).

Wahlstrom also summarized key results from surveys conducted with more than 7,000 students in three Minnesota school districts, using the Brown University School Sleep Habits Survey. The main purpose was to discover any differences among students in one district that had changed to a later starting time and two others in which the earlier starting time was maintained. Researchers found significant differences in students' responses regarding their sleep habits. Where the later time was instituted, students reported getting a full hour more of sleep than those with the earlier starting time. These students also reported less overall sleepiness, less daytime sleepiness, and less depression, as well as higher grades than their peers in the other schools. These findings do not indicate causality—that a later starting time will cause improvement in academic grades—but do show a statistical relationship between these two variables that may be explained by such things as less struggle to stay awake in class when starting times are later.

Attitudes Toward School Starting and Dismissal Times

To shed light on how teachers and other school professionals view current starting and dismissal times, researchers also surveyed more than 3,000 secondary school teachers. More than half of the high school teachers surveyed said the optimal time to start school is 8:00 a.m. or later. When asked what would be the latest time to end the instructional day without negative impact on such activities as sports, debate club, or choir, almost 44 percent said that a 3:00 p.m. dismissal time would not have a negative impact on these activities.

A telephone survey of 765 parents included a question about preferred time for their children to leave home in the morning. For senior high school students, most parents preferred a time of 8:00 a.m. Forty-five percent said they gave that reason because it allows more sleep.

Workshop participants emphasized that later school starting times are not a panacea for adolescent sleep problems, nor do they work well for all students or all school districts. Regardless of what time school starts, some adolescents may need to get up earlier to take care of siblings or to get a ride to school. For those considering such a change, it is essential to glean data from sleep research. Armed with the available knowledge, school boards and communities can have an informed debate. Any change in education systems requires gathering all stakeholders to review the data and debate the range of possible options. Public awareness and education also are crucial, as is the involvement of key education officials.

EDUCATING THE PUBLIC ABOUT
ADOLESCENT SLEEP NEEDS

Workshop participants agreed that the issue of helping adolescents get more sleep is complex. Several identified a need for the public to be better informed about the biological (circadian and homeostatic) influences on adolescent sleep patterns. At the same time, social and behavioral influences play a critical role and need to be recognized. In the laboratory or another setting, such as a camping trip, it is possible to strip away such distractions as television, computers, phones, social events, and lights, and adolescents are more likely to go to sleep early and get up early, getting their required amount of sleep without problems. But returning to society, current cultural influences, and their own habits, they revert to the sleeping patterns that have been documented as causing problems. How can more informed practices be developed? Workshop participants looked at public education and social marketing approaches that have had positive effects in other public health areas.

Lloyd Kolbe, director of the Division of Adolescent and School Health at the Centers for Disease Control and Prevention, discussed the public health perspective, with its focus on treatment and prevention. These approaches attempt to change not only the population at risk—young people—but also the societal institutions that most influence their health and development. Public health approaches are necessarily long term and gain synergy from cooperation and collaboration. Changing existing cultural norms around teenagers' sleep behaviors probably will require a decade-long effort. More than a single institution, whether that be schools or health care providers, must be involved. Each of these institutions faces competing demands—improving SAT scores, coping with the HIV (human immunodeficiency virus) epidemic, or drug and alcohol use—that require attention.

Successful efforts to change attitudes and behaviors, Kolbe said, would be based on population-based data on educational or health outcomes, increases in productivity, decreases in impulsivity, and other conclusions from studies of adolescent sleep, such as those presented at the workshop. The financial and practical implications of implementing changes also need to be spelled out.

To avoid patchwork approaches, it may be useful to think about addressing the issue simultaneously from the local, state, and national perspectives. This would tap the creativity and communication channels of both government and the private sector (see Boxes 3 and 4). The array of institutions and groups is very broad: parents and families; schools, including teachers and their organizations, school counselors and psychologists, school administrators and superintendents; health care professionals, including physicians and nurses and their associations, such as the American Academy of Pediatrics and the Society for Adolescent Medicine; businesses that employ youth; and higher education, including medical schools, schools of public health, colleges of education, and schools of government and public affairs. Government has a critical role to play, as U.S. Representative Zoe Lofgren discussed at the workshop (see Box 5). Particularly important are state legislatures, especially on issues of education. With the necessary leadership to bring these and other key stakeholders together, it may be possible to bring about more coherent and comprehensive change than could be achieved one school at a time or one district at a time.

NEXT STEPS

Workshop participants agreed that raising public and professional awareness of the sleep needs of adolescents and the consequences of insufficient sleep is critical. Research findings presented at the workshop on the effects of inadequate sleep on mood, academic and work performance, physical and mental health, and traffic safety are compelling but need to be more widely known among policy makers, parents, young people, and the public. According to a poll conducted by the National Sleep Foundation,

---

BOX 3 Getting the Word Out

"Back to Sleep" Campaign

One of the most successful public health campaigns of the past decade is the "Back to Sleep" campaign carried out in this country and throughout the developed world to help prevent sudden infant death syndrome (SIDS). Marian Willinger, special assistant for sudden infant death syndrome at the National Institute on Child Health and Human Development (NICHD), reported on the campaign's evolution, planning, and implementation. In contrast to concerns about adolescent sleep, both the medical community and the public were generally aware of the risk of SIDS. Several population-based studies had been carried out, revealing a strong association between infants' sleeping on their stomachs and the incidence of SIDS. With the impetus of the American Academy of Pediatrics Task Force on Infant Positioning and Sudden Infant Death as well as continuing research by NICHD and others in this country and abroad showing promising results, especially overseas, a coalition of the medical community, parents' advocacy organizations, and state-level alliances initiated the public education campaign. The message was simple, a catchy phrase was selected—"Back to Sleep"—based on a similar British campaign, and a public service announcement campaign was launched. Target audiences were chosen, and dissemination of materials to parents, hospitals, and day care providers was free and widespread. Evaluations of the campaign indicate a high level of impact on public awareness and on behavior.

---

most Americans get less sleep than they need, with 30 percent usually sleeping 6.5 hours a night or less during the work week; 40 percent report that daytime sleepiness interferes with their daily activities. More than 60 percent have driven while feeling drowsy, and 27 percent report that they have dozed off while driving, if only for a moment. This poll also found that 60 percent of children complained to their parents about being tired. Nearly a quarter of parents with children living at home and 23 percent of adults without children favor later school starting times (National Sleep Foundation, 1999).

Workshop participants noted the complexities involved in changing awareness and understanding of sleep needs in a culture in which high

---

BOX 4 Getting the Message into the Media

Another approach taken by organizations that seek to raise awareness of a problem and change behavior is the National Campaign to Prevent Teen Pregnancy, which was launched in 1997. One of its key approaches is working with the media. The campaign has developed partnerships with people in the entertainment industry to help them reach audiences with messages about teen pregnancy prevention.

Sarah Brown, campaign director, discussed issues relating to whether and how to engage the mass entertainment media—television, radio, magazines—in conveying important health information. The campaign always begins with the facts, drawing on the best science and research, and reaching out to include key stakeholders, including parents, schools, the faith community, business, and teens themselves. In developing their media program, they recognized that the impact of media messages in changing behavior is still not clear. Research on public service announcements, for example, indicates that kids tune these out. So the campaign focuses on engaging media leaders as partners and friends. The approach involves getting messages into the story lines of entertainment programs and media that reach the target audience. The campaign offers a range of messages that are based on research; the choice to use them is, of course, up to the media. To date, the campaign has been successful in getting messages in such magazines as *Teen People*, the story line of such television programs as ABC's "One Life to Live" and Black Entertainment Television's "Teen Summit" series.

---

levels of activity and extended work schedules symbolize success. Similarly, young people themselves deal with the distractions of social life and entertainment media that impinge on their sleep. In the policy arena, consideration of such issues as changes in school starting times must compete against very real concerns about the financial implications, the impact on the variety of reform efforts, and the effect on extracurricular activities seen as important to strengthening adolescents' connection to their schools.

A starting point for both education and policy analysis is the science behind adolescent sleep needs and difficulties. While time and other constraints at the workshop limited the amount of detailed information presented, the wealth of research available is suggested by both the references

---

BOX 5 The Zzzzz's to A's Act

Workshop participants also learned of one policy maker's response to concerns about adolescent sleep. Representative Zoe Lofgren (D-CA) reported that she had introduced legislation to provide a small amount of funds to encourage school districts to consider whether school starting times should be changed. Known as the "Zzzzz's to A's Act," the bill was proposed in March 1999 in conjunction with National Sleep Awareness Week. The legislation would make it easier for high schools to cover the increased operating costs associated with changing school starting times by providing up to $25,000. Prominent researchers, including those present at the workshop, have endorsed the bill.

Representative Lofgren acknowledged that the money would simply be an incentive rather than funding for all the costs involved. She also candidly acknowledged that her bill stands little chance of passing. However, the bill officially recognizes what researchers, parents, and teachers know: high school students are suffering from sleep loss while trying to cope with the stresses of school, work, and social activities. She called experiences in jurisdictions that have tried later starting times promising.

She also noted the "morality" issue that comes into play when discussing adolescents and sleep that is not present in looking at other problems. As other participants noted, sleepiness is seen as a character defect. She urged that science-based information on the effects of inadequate sleep on learning, academic achievement, and accidents be brought to the attention of school boards.

---

and the sources for additional information that appear at the end of this report. Greater awareness and understanding of this research can help parents, teachers, and teens themselves see the problem from a different perspective.

Participants noted that additional research on young people would help to both disentangle the factors contributing to adolescent sleep problems and assess their long-term effects. In particular, more documentation of sleep debt and its size in high school students is needed, comparing students without a sleep debt to those with a large sleep debt. More in-depth studies also should focus on the perspective of teens themselves on their sleep habits and problems. Other questions for research include the following:

- How can we better understand the sensitivity of the circadian system to changes in ambient light?
- Would providing bright light in the morning in homes and schools help students who are drowsy?
- What is the parental role in monitoring adolescents' sleep schedules in both the United States and other countries?
- What are the contextual and cultural issues related to sleep that require investigation?
- How can more complete and methodologically sound comparisons be drawn between adolescent sleep patterns in the United States and those in other industrialized countries?
- What are the costs and benefits of measures to counter the problem of inadequate adolescent sleep?

As research on these and other important questions continues, the growing knowledge should be applied to designing interventions that promote better sleep habits and improve the health and safety of adolescents. These include more effective identification of sleep problems in young people and approaches for reducing automobile accidents caused by drowsy drivers. Similarly, broad dissemination of research findings is essential. As workshop participants noted, such communication efforts could draw on a variety of disciplines and organizations that have a stake in understanding adolescent sleep difficulties and possible approaches to help young people, their families, their schools, and the health care system promote healthy adolescent development.

References

Andrade, M.M., E.E. Benedito-Silva, and S. Domenice
  1993 Sleep characteristics of adolescents: A longitudinal study. *Journal of Adolescent Health* 14:401-406.
Carskadon, M.A.
  1982 The second decade. Pp. 99-125 in C. Guilleminault, ed. *Sleeping and Waking Disorders: Indications and Techniques.* Menlo Park, CA: Addison Wesley.
  1990 Patterns of sleep and sleepiness in adolescents. *Pediatrician* 17:5-12.
Carskadon, M.A., and W.C. Dement
  1981 Cumulative effects of sleep restriction on daytime sleepiness. *The Society for Psychophysiological Research* 18(2):107-113.
Carskadon, M.A., K. Harvey, P. Duke, T.F. Anders, I.F. Litt, and W.C. Dement
  1980 Pubertal changes in daytime sleepiness. *Sleep* 2:453-460.
Carskadon, M.A., W.C. Dement, M.M. Mitler, T. Roth, P. Westbrook, and S. Keenan
  1986 Guidelines for the Multiple Sleep Latency Test (MSLT): A standard measure of sleepiness. *Sleep* 9:519-524.
Carskadon, M.A., A.R. Wolfson, C. Acebo, O. Tzischinsky, and R. Safer
  1998 Circadian timing and sleepiness at a transition to early school days. *Sleep* 21(8): 871-881.
Carskadon, M.A., S.E. Labyak, C. Acebo, and R. Seifer
  1999 Intrinsic circadian period of adolescent humans measured in conditions of forced desynchrony. *Neuroscience Letters* 260:129-132.
Dahl, R.E.
  1999 The consequences of insufficient sleep for adolescents: Links between sleep and emotional regulation. *Kappan* 80(5):354-359.
Dahl, R.E., et al.
  1996 Sleep onset abnormalities in depressed adolescents. *Biological Psychiatry* 39:400-410.

31

Dahl, R.E., J. Hotturn, and L. Trubnick
    1994   A clinical picture of child and adolescent narcolepsy. *Journal of the American Academy of Adolescent Psychiatry* 33:834-841.
Dinges, D.
    1995   An overview of sleepiness and accidents in drowsy driving. *Journal of Sleep Research* 4(2):4-14.
Dinges, D., et al.
    1997   Cumulative sleepiness, mood disturbance, and psychomotor vigilance performance during a week of sleep restricted to 4-5 hours per night. *Sleep* 20(4):267-277.
Elster, A.B., and N.J. Kuznets
    1993   *AMA Guidelines for Adolescent Preventive Services (GAPS).* Chicago: American Medical Association.
Gau, S.F., and W.T. Soong
    1995   Sleep problems of junior high school students in Taipei: Pediatric sleep disorders. *Sleep* 18(8):667-673.
Hofman, W.F., and L. Steenhof
    1998   Sleep characteristics of Dutch adolescents and the relation with school performance. *Sleep-Wake Research in the Netherlands* 8:51-55.
Knipling, R.R., and J. Wang
    1995   Revised estimates of the U.S. drowsy driver crash problem size based on general estimates system case reviews. Pp. 451-466 in *Thirty-Ninth Annual Proceedings of the Association for the Advancement of Automotive Medicine.* Chicago, Illinois.
Kubow, P., K. Wahlstrom, and A. Bemis
    1999   Starting Time and School Life. *Kappan* 80(5):344-347.
Lands, W.E.
    1999   Alcohol, slow-wave sleep, and the somatotropic axis. *Alcohol* 18(2-3):109-122.
Minors, D.S., J.M. Waterhouse, and A. Wirz-Justice
    1991   A human phase response curve to light. *Neuroscience Letters* 133:36-40.
Mortimer, J.T., C. Harley, and P.J. Anderson
    1999   How do prior experiences in the workplace set the stage for transitions to adulthood? Pp. 131-159 in *Transition to Adulthood in a Changing Economy.* Westport, CT: Praeger.
National Highway Traffic Safety Administration
    1999   *Fatality Analysis Reporting System (FARS) 1995-1998.* "Drowsy" Drivers Involved in Fatal Crashes, by Sex and Age (Driver related factor of drowsy, sleepy, asleep, or fatigued). Washington, D.C.: U.S. Department of Transportation.
National Research Council and Institute of Medicine
    1999   *Adolescent Development and the Biology of Puberty: Summary of a Workshop on New Research.* Forum on Adolescence, Michele D. Kipke, ed. Board on Children, Youth, and Families, Commission on Behavioral and Social Sciences and Education. Washington, D.C.: National Academy Press.
    1998   *Adolescent Decision Making: Implications for Prevention Programs. Summary of a Workshop.* Board on Children, Youth, and Families, Baruch Fischhoff, Nancy A. Crowell, and Michele D. Kipke, eds. Commission on Behavioral and Social Sciences and Education. Washington, D.C.: National Academy Press.

National Sleep Foundation
   1999   *Omnibus Sleep in America Poll.* Washington, D.C.: National Sleep Foundation.
Pack, A., et al.
   1995   Characteristics of crashes attributed to the driver having fallen asleep. *Accident Analysis and Prevention* 27(6):769-775.
Phillips, B.A., and F.J. Danner
   1995   Cigarette smoking and sleep disturbance. *Archives of Internal Medicine* 155: 734-737.
Schoen, C., K. Davis, K. Collins, L. Greenberg, et al.
   1997   *The Commonwealth Fund Survey of the Health of Adolescent Girls.* New York: Louis Harris and Associates, Inc.
Tynjala, J., L. Kannas, and R. Vailimaa
   1993   How young Europeans sleep? *Health Education Research* 8:69-80.
Vignau, J., D. Bailly, A. Duhamel, P. Vervaecke, R. Beuscart, and C. Collinet
   1997   Epidemiologic study of sleep quality and troubles in French secondary school adolescents. *Journal of Adolescent Health* 21:343-350.
Wahlstrom, K.L.
   1997   *School Start Time Study: Technical Report, Volume II: Analysis of Student Survey Data.* Minneapolis, MN: Center for Applied Research and Educational Improvement.
   1999   The prickly politics of school starting times. *Kappan* 80(5):344-347.
Wahlstrom, K.L., and C.M. Freeman
   1997   *School Start Time Study: Preliminary Report of Findings.* Minneapolis, MN: Center for Applied Research and Educational Improvement.
Wang, J., R. Knipling, and M. Goodman
   1996   The role of driver inattention in crashes: New statistics from the 1995 crashworthiness data system. Pp. 377-392 in *Fortieth Annual Proceedings of the Association for the Advancement of Automotive Medicine.* Vancouver, British Columbia.
Winkelman, J.W.
   1998   Clinical and polysomnographic features of sleep-related eating disorder. *Journal of Clinical Psychiatry* 59:14-19.
Wolfson, A.R.
   in   Bridging the gap between research and practice: What will adolescents' sleep/
   press   wake patterns look like in the 21st century? In M.A. Carskadon, ed., *Adolescent Sleep Patterns: Biological, Social and Psychological Influences.* New York: Cambridge University Press.
Wolfson, A.R., and M.A. Carskadon
   1998   Sleep schedules and daytime functioning in adolescents. *Child Development* 69(4):875-887.

OTHER INFORMATION RESOURCES

American Academy of Sleep Medicine
6301 Bandel Road, NW
Suite 101
Rochester, MN 55901
507-287-6006
507-287-6008 (fax)
aasm@aasmnet.org
http://www.aasmnet.org

National Center on Sleep Disorders Research
NIH/NHLBI/NCSDR
Two Rockledge Centre Suite 10038
6701 Rockledge Drive MSC 7920
Bethesda, MD 20892-7920
301-435-0199
301-480-3451 (fax)
ncsdr@nih.gov
http://www.nhlbi.nih.gov/about/ncsdr

National Sleep Foundation
1522 K Street, NW
Suite 500
Washington, DC 20005
202-347-3471
202-347-3472 (fax)
natsleep@erols.com
http://www.sleepfoundation.org/about.html

Appendix

Workshop Agenda and Participants

Workshop on the Sleep Needs, Patterns, and
Difficulties of Adolescents

Forum on Adolescence
Board on Children, Youth, and Families

Wednesday, September 22, 1999

Location: National Academy of Sciences
Lecture Room
2101 Constitution Avenue, NW
Washington, D.C. 20418

8:30-9:00   Continental Breakfast

9:00-9:30   **Orientation to the Meeting and Recent History of
                 Sleep Research**

                 David A. Hamburg (Workshop Cochair)
                 Chair, Forum on Adolescence

                 William C. Dement (Workshop Cochair)
                 Director, Sleep Disorders Center
                 Stanford University

9:30-9:55   **The Zzz's to A's Legislation**
                   The Honorable Zoe Lofgren (D-CA)
                   U.S. House of Representatives

                   Questions and Answers

9:55-10:20   **Understanding and Meeting the Developmental Needs**
                   of Adolescents

                   Adolescent Development: Individual and Contextual
                   Considerations
                   Robert Blum
                   Professor and Director
                   Division of General Pediatrics and Adolescent Health,
                   Department of Pediatrics
                   University of Minnesota

                   Questions and Answers

10:20-11:20   Research on the Sleep Needs and Difficulties of
                   Adolescents

                   Adolescent Sleep: The Transition from Early to Bed Early to
                   Rise to Too Little Too Late
                   Mary Carskadon
                   Director, Chronobiology and Sleep Research Laboratory
                   Brown University

                   International Comparison of Adolescent Sleep Patterns
                   Amy Wolfson
                   Associate Professor, Department of Psychology
                   College of the Holy Cross
                   Worcester, Massachusetts

                   Questions and Answers

11:20-11:35   Break

11:35-12:30   **Consequences of Insufficient Sleep and Sleep Difficulties**

Insufficient Sleep in Adolescence: Effects on Mood, Attention, and Social Competence
Ronald Dahl
Director, Child and Adolescent Sleep Evaluation Center
University of Pittsburgh Medical Center

Neurobehavioral Effects of Chronic Sleep Restrictions
David Dinges
Chief, Division of Sleep and Chronobiology
University of Pennsylvania

Discussant: Russell Poland
Professor, Department of Psychiatry & Biobehavioral Sciences
Harbor-UCLA Medical Center

Questions and Answers

12:30-1:30   **Working Lunch**

National Sleep Foundation's Sleep and Teens Task Force
Richard Gelula
Executive Director, National Sleep Foundation

1:30-2:15   **Redesigning the Day to Meet the Developmental and Sleep Needs of Teens**

Working and Adolescent Development
Jeylan Mortimer
Professor, Department of Sociology
University of Minnesota

Later School Start Time Research: Policies, Politics, and Preliminary Outcomes
Kyla Wahlstrom
Associate Director, Center for Applied Research and Educational Improvement
University of Minnesota

Discussant: Richard Ferber
               Director, Center for Pediatric Sleep Disorders
               Children's Hospital, Boston

Questions and Answers

2:15-3:15   **Identifying and Intervening in Sleep Problems**

Teenagers and Sleep Deprivation: The View from a Teacher and Mother
Cathy Colglaizer
Teacher, English Department
McLean High School
Fairfax County Public Schools

The Ephebiatrician's View of the Sleepy Teenager
Iris Litt
Director, Division of Adolescent Medicine
Stanford University

Identifying and Intervening in Sleep Problems: A Clinician's Perspective
Mark Mahowald
Director, Minnesota Regional Sleep Disorders Center
Hennepin County Medical Center

Discussant: Lloyd Kolbe
               Director, Division of Adolescent and School Health
               Centers for Disease Control and Prevention

Questions and Answers

3:15-4:00   **Increasing Public Awareness of and Interest in Adolescents' Sleep and Developmental Needs**

National Public Education Campaign: "Back to Sleep"
Marian Willinger
Special Assistant for Sudden Infant Death Syndrome
National Institute on Child Health and Human Development

Getting Messages into the Media
Sarah Brown
Director, National Campaign to Prevent Teen Pregnancy

Questions and Answers

4:00-4:25   **Looking to the Future: Integrating Research, Policy, and Practice**

William C. Dement
Workshop Chair

4:25-4:30   **Closing Remarks**

Michele D. Kipke
Director, Board on Children, Youth, and Families

4:30   **Adjourn**

PARTICIPANTS

CHRISTINE ACEBO, E.P. Bradley Hospital, Brown University School of Medicine

RICHARD P. ALLEN, PLS Medical Advisory Board, Johns Hopkins Sleep Disorder Center, Arnold, Maryland

EVVIE BECKER, Office of the Assistant Secretary for Planning and Evaluation, U.S. Department of Health and Human Services

JESSE BLATT, Office of Research and Traffic Records, National Highway Traffic Safety Administration, U.S. Department of Transportation, Washington, D.C.

ROBERT BLUM, Division of General Pediatrics and Adolescent Health, University of Minnesota Medical School

WINSLOW J. BORKOWSKI, JR., Thomas Jefferson Medical School, Dupont Children's Hospital, Wilmington, Delaware

KIERSTAN BOYD, National Science Foundation, Washington, D.C.

JAMES BREILING, Violence and Traumatic Stress Research, National Institute of Mental Health, U.S. Department of Health and Human Services

PAT BRITZ, National Science Foundation, Washington, D.C.

BARBARA BRODY, Driver Education Improvement, St. Cloud State University

SARAH BROWN, National Campaign to Prevent Teenage Pregnancy, Washington, D.C.

MARY M. CAMPBELL, Public Interest Directorate, American Psychological Association, Washington, D.C.

MARY CARSKADON, Chronobiology and Sleep Research Laboratory, E.P. Bradley Hospital, Brown University School of Medicine

JANET CHAPIN, Division of Women's Health Issues, American College of Obstetricians and Gynecologists, Washington, D.C.

SONIA G. CHESSEN, Human Services Policy, Office of the Assistant Secretary for Planning and Evaluation, U.S. Department of Health and Human Services, Washington, D.C.

CATHERINE COLGLAZIER, English Department, McLean High School, McLean, Virginia

RONALD DAHL, Psychiatry and Pediatrics, Director, Child and Adolescent Sleep Evaluation Center, University of Pittsburgh Medical Center

WILLIAM DEMENT, Department of Psychiatry, Director, Sleep
Disorders Center, Stanford University

CYNTHIA DIEHM, National Clearinghouse on Families and Youth,
U.S. Department of Health and Human Services

DAVID DINGES, Division of Sleep and Chronobiology, University of
Pennsylvania, School of Medicine

DARREL DROBNICH, National Sleep Foundation, Washington, D.C.

CHERYL A. DUKES, National Medical Association, Washington, D.C.

CHRISTIAN ENGELHARAT, American Sleep Apnea Association,
Washington, D.C.

STEPHANIE FAUL, American Automobile Association Foundation for
Traffic Safety, Washington, D.C.

MARGARET FELDMAN, National Council on Family Relations,
Washington, D.C.

RICHARD FERBER, Center for Pediatric Sleep Disorders, Children's
Hospital, Boston, Massachusetts

ROLAND W. FINKEN, Virginia Coordinator for A.W.A.K.E., and
Chair, Fairfax County Public Schools, Later Starting Times
Committee, NSF/ASAA/Wake Up America, McLean, Virginia

ANNABELLE FISHER, Center for Child Protection and Family
Support, Washington, D.C.

MICHAEL FISHMAN, Division of Child, Adolescent, and Family
Health, MCHB, Rockville, Maryland

PATRICIA B. FLYNN, Department of Academic Programs,
Montgomery County Public Schools, Rockville, Maryland

BRIDGET FREEMAN, Healthy Adolescents Project, Public Interest
Directorate, American Psychological Association, Washington, D.C.

YVONNE FULLER, National Medical Association, Washington, D.C.

RALPH GALLO, University Services Sleep Labs, Wynnewood,
Pennsylvania

RICHARD GELULA, National Sleep Foundation, Washington, D.C.

CHARLETA GUILLORY, Baylor College of Medicine, Texas Children's
Hospital, Houston, Texas

DAVID HAMBURG, Carnegie Corporation of New York, New York

PAMELA HAMILTON-STUBBS, Richmond, Virginia

ISADORA R. HARE, Healthy Adolescents Project, Public Interest
Directorate, American Psychological Association, Washington, D.C.

GREGORY HARPER, Comprehensive Sleep TX, Alexandria, Virginia

JAMES C. HARRIS, Developmental Neuropsychiatry, School of Medicine, Johns Hopkins University

LYNNE HAVERKOS, Research Programs in Behavioral Pediatrics and Health Promotion, National Institute of Child Health and Human Development

KARIN F. HELMERS, National Institute of Nursing Research, National Institutes of Health, U.S. Department of Health and Human Services

DAVID HEPPEL, Division of Maternal, Infant, Child, and Adolescent Health, Health Resources and Service Administration, U.S. Department of Health and Human Services

CHERYL HOLMES, College of Social Work, University of Tennessee

IRENE KARALIS, Bethesda, Maryland

MARIANA KASTRINAKIS, Office of the Deputy Assistant Secretary for Population Affairs, U.S. Department of Health and Human Services

FRANCIS C. KENEL, American Driver and Traffic Safety Education Association, American Automobile Association, Silver Spring, Maryland

JAMES P. KILEY, National Center on Sleep Disorders Research, National Institutes of Health, Bethesda, Maryland

LLOYD KOLBE, Division of Adolescent and School Health, Centers for Disease Control and Prevention, Atlanta, Georgia

NANCY KOPF, Department of Educational Accountability, Montgomery County Public Schools, Rockville, Maryland

SURESH KOTAGAL, St. Louis University Health Sciences Center, St. Louis, Missouri

ISREAL I. LEDERHENDLER, National Institute of Mental Health, National Institutes of Health

IRIS LITT, Division of Adolescent Medicine, Stanford University School of Medicine

ZOE LOFGREN, Working Group on Children, U.S. House of Representatives, Washington, D.C.

JEFFREY P. LUCAS, The Nation's Health and American Public Health Association, Washington, D.C.

TERRI LUKAS, PTSA Bethesda-Chevy Chase, Maryland

MARK MAHOWALD, Minnesota Regional Sleep Disorders Center, Hennepin County Medical Center, Minneapolis, Minnesota

ISABELLE MELESE-D'HOSPITAL, EMSC National Resource Center, Silver Spring, Maryland

SUSAN-MARIE MARSH, OSERS/OSEP, Washington, D.C.

JAMES T. McCRACKEN, Division of Child and Adolescent Psychiatry, UCLA Neuropsychiatric Institute

PAMELA A. McCULLOUGH, Sleep Medicine Specialists, Louisville, Kentucky

WILLIAM MODZELESKI, Safe and Drug-Free Schools Program, Office of Elementary and Secondary Education, U.S. Department of Education

JEYLAN MORTIMER, Department of Sociology, University of Minnesota

JEANNINE NIELSEN, Office of Population Affairs, U.S. Department of Health and Human Services

EDITHA NOTTLEMANN, Depression, Anxiety, and Regulatory Disorders Program, National Institute of Mental Health, U.S. Department of Health and Human Services

EDWARD O'MALLEY, NH Sleep Disorders Center, New York University School of Medicine, Norwalk Hospital Sleep Disorders Center, Norwalk, Connecticut

MARK OUELETTE, National Governor's Association, Washington, D.C.

AVERETTE PARKER, Office of Minority Health Concerns, U.S. Department of Health and Human Services, Rockville, Maryland

JOANNA PARZAKONIS, American Academy of Pediatrics, Washington, D.C.

ALBERT A. PAWLOWSKI, Alcohol Medical Research Foundation, Baltimore, Maryland

PHILLIP L. PEARL, Children's National Medical Center, Washington, D.C.

LUCILE PEREZ, Center for Substance Abuse Prevention, National Medical Association, Rockville, Maryland

JAMES R. PERLSTROM, Greater Washington Sleep Disorders Center, Rockville, Maryland

LETITIA PIERCE, Towson, Maryland

RUSSELL POLAND, Harbor-UCLA Medical Center, Torrance, California

BONNIE POLITZ, Center for Youth Development and Policy Research, Academy for Educational Development, Washington, D.C.

ANGELA RENDAZZO, Sleep Medicine Research, Chesterfield, Missouri

MARSHA RENWANZ, COSSHMO, Washington, D.C.

ANITA ROBINSON, Department of Pediatrics, National Naval Medical Center, Bethesda, Maryland

GLEN E. ROBINSON, Educational Research Service, Bethesda, Maryland

SUE ROGUS, Sleep Education Activities, National Center on Sleep Disorders Research, National Institutes of Health, U.S Department of Health and Human Services

AVI SADEH, Children's Sleep Laboratory, Department of Psychology, Tel-Aviv University, Ramat Aviv, Israel

SUSAN SAGUSTI, National Sleep Foundation, Washington, D.C.

NANCY SCONYERS, National Association of Child Advocates, Washington, D.C.

LAURA SESSIONS STEPP, The Washington *Post*, Washington, D.C.

THERESA SHUMARD, Association of Polysomnographic Technologists, Mohnton, Pennsylvania

MONA SIGNER, Montgomery County Board of Education, Rockville, Maryland

PHILLIP L. SMITH, Indian Health Center, Rockville, Maryland

KINGMAN STROHL, Case Western Reserve University

DEBRA VIADERO, *Education Week*, Bethesda, Maryland

KYLA WAHLSTROM, Center for Applied Research and Educational Improvement, University of Minnesota

RICHARD WALDHORN, Sleep Disorders Center, Georgetown University Medical Center

JOYCE WALSLEBEN, New York University Sleep Disorders Center, New York University School of Medicine

ELIZABETH WEHR, Center for Health Policy Research, George Washington University Medical Center

PATIENCE H. WHITE, Adolescent Employment Readiness Center, Pediatric Rheumatology, Children's National Medical Center, Washington, D.C.

SHERYL WILLIAMS, Cephalon, Westchester, Pennsylvania

MARIAN WILLINGER, Special Assistant for Sudden Infant Death Syndrome, National Institute on Child Health and Human Development, National Institutes of Health, U.S Department of Health and Human Services

DAVID K. WILLIS, American Automobile Association Foundation for Traffic Safety, Washington, D.C.

AMY WOLFSON, Department of Psychology, College of the Holy Cross

CAROL M. WORTHMAN, Department of Anthropology,
Emory University
HELEN I. YOUNGMAN, Maryland School-Based Health Center
Initiative, Governor's Office for Children, Youth, and Families,
Baltimore, Maryland
DIANA ZUCKERMAN, Institute for Women's Policy Research,
Washington, D.C.

Selected Reports of the Board on Children, Youth, and Families

After-School Programs to Promote Child and Adolescent Development: Summary of a Workshop (2000)

Early Childhood Intervention: Views from the Field. Report of a Workshop (2000)

Improving Intergroup Relations Among Youth: Summary of a Research Workshop (2000)

Risks and Opportunities: Synthesis of Studies on Adolescence (1999)

Adolescent Development and the Biology of Puberty: Summary of a Workshop on New Research (1999)

Adolescent Decision Making: Implications for Prevention Programs: Summary of a Workshop (1999)

Revisiting Home Visiting: Summary of a Workshop (1999)

Protecting Youth at Work: Health, Safety, and Development of Working Children and Adolescents in the United States (1998)

America's Children: Health Insurance and Access to Care (with the IOM Division of Health Care Services; 1998)

Systems of Accountability: Implementing Children's Health Insurance Programs (with the IOM Division of Health Care Services; 1998)

Longitudinal Surveys of Children: Report of a Workshop (with the NRC Committee on National Statistics; 1998)

From Generation to Generation: The Health and Well-Being of Children in Immigrant Families (1998)

New Findings on Poverty and Child Health and Nutrition: Summary of a Research Briefing (1998)

Violence in Families: Assessing Treatment and Prevention Programs (1998)

Welfare, the Family, and Reproductive Behavior: Report of a Meeting (with the NRC Committee on Population; 1998)

Educating Language-Minority Children (1998)

Improving Schooling for Language-Minority Children: A Research Agenda (1997)

New Findings on Welfare and Children's Development: Summary of a Research Briefing (1997)

Youth Development and Neighborhood Influences: Challenges and Opportunities: Summary of a Workshop (1996)

Paying Attention to Children in a Changing Health Care System: Summaries of Workshops (1996)

Integrating Federal Statistics on Children (with the NRC Committee on National Statistics; 1995)